The Accessible Games Book

of related interest

Helping Children to Build Self-Esteem
A Photocopiable Activities Book
Deborah Plummer
ISBN 1 85302 927 0

Growing Up With Disability
Edited by Carol Robinson and Kirsten Stalker
ISBN 1 85302 568 2

Housing Options for Disabled People
Edited by Ruth Bull
Preface by Baroness Masham
ISBN 1 85302 454 6

The Accessible Games Book

Collated and Adapted by Katie Marl

Jessica Kingsley Publishers
London and Philadelphia

First published in the United Kingdom in 1996

This edition published in 1999 by
Jessica Kingsley Publishers
116 Pentonville Road
London, N1 9JB, UK

and

400 Market Street, Suite 400
Philadelphia PA 19106, USA

www.jkp.com

Copyright ©1996, 1999 Katie Marl
Printed digitally since 2004

Library of Congress Cataloging in Publication Data

Marl, Katie, 1974–
    The accessible games book / Katie Marl.
        p.   cm.
    Includes index.
    ISBN 1-85302-830-4 (pbk. : alk. paper)
    1. Hadicapped children--Recreation. 2. Handicapped--Recreation. 3. Educational games. I. Title.
LC4026.M37 1999
790. 2'96--dc21   99-43194

British Library Cataloguing in Publication Data

A CIP catalogue record for this book is available from the British Library

ISBN 1 85302 830 4

Introduction

Increasingly, people with disabilities can be seen more frequently in community, education and work settings. This book has come about from a belief that when companies, playschemes, schools or conferences use games to integrate people and to promote mixing, this aim can only be achieved if the games are accessible. Games that are *not* accessible only highlight to everyone the ability levels we each have.

The games I have included may well be familiar to you, but I have sought to adapt them so that they are accessible to a greater number of people, particularly those with disabilities. Games are classified as suitable for small groups (under 10), medium groups (10–40) and large groups (40+), but please remember the small or medium group games could be appropriate to a larger group which has been sub-divided. At the end, everyone could gather for a whole group discussion or feedback session. I have also indicated if I think the games are useful as a disability awareness raising exercise.

The book is divided into sections which include the most suitable games for each level of ability. However, this classification is only a starting point – most games can be played with most groups of players, and groups should be adventurous in the games they choose. For further classification, symbols have been used to show which particular abilities are necessary for some games. The symbols I have used are as follows:

indicating that sight is required

 indicating that hearing is required (if this sign is not present it presumes that profoundly deaf people have interpreters in order to take part, for instructions etc.)

 indicating that upper body strength and mobility, and co-ordination is required

 indicating that mobility is required.

Equally as important as these symbols are the variations and comments written below the game procedures which provide advice on how to make them more accessible. In some cases these variations make the game accessible to a client group for whom it may not initially have seemed appropriate.

Further points you should think about when making games accessible include:

★ Always ensure there is enough scope in the options you provide for people to work at their own level; for example, instead of giving the instruction 'go to the door in the style of a frog', say 'go to your left in the style of an animal'. That way people choose an animal they can physically portray in action and sound, and move the distance they can manage. Also, giving open directions such as 'move to the left...' means blind people can more easily take part, and people are spread out more evenly. This reduces congestion and obvious distinctions between fast and slow movers.

★ If games involve moving around the room while making arm movements, wheelchair users are automatically excluded – they can't drive! Action must be something simple like nodding the head.

★ Place chairs around the room to allow people with walking difficulties to sit at certain stages in the game.

★ Describing what will happen in the game to the group before starting allows disabled players to assess the suitability for them, and allows for preparation from one stage of the game to another; for example, people with walking difficulties can move to the part of the hall where they know they need to be next.

★ Don't play games that involve the group mirroring actions of one person – this makes a person's limitations obvious.

★ If written sheets are to be used during the game (e.g. in Human Bingo) copies with print blown up to at least 24pt should be available for those with sight difficulties.

It is hoped that this book will become a working document. Comments on the suitability of games, further suggestions to aid accessibility and more accessible games would be gratefully received. You can contact me through my publishers.

My thanks go to: all those who suggested and provided games to be used, including:

SCADU and the SCA network
Ali, Alison, Tasha and Michelle for helping me with the planning and collating
West Lancashire Association of Disabled People and Edge Hill University
College for their financial backing and support of the research for this book.
Mikey for all his computer fiddling
Julie for her brilliant suitability illustrations
Vics for the front cover illustration
and all the other people who supported me while writing this book.

Good luck using the book, and enjoy providing fun for EVERYONE!

Contents

Introductory games

Clapping Names

Group size: Medium / Large

Procedure

1 Everyone sits in a circle.

2 The group practise clapping a rhythm, but with a gap in it (eg. clap, clap, rest).

3 Taking turns round the circle, each player should call out their name in the gap.

4 Next time around, each player should call out the name of the person next to him/her in the gap.

Variations

★ Players call out their own name and then the name of anyone else in the circle. It now becomes his/her turn and s/he has to do the same thing in the next gap.

Comments

★ The ability of individuals to maintain the clapping is not evident if the group size is large enough.

Collecting Names

Group size: Medium

Procedure

1   Everyone sits in a circle.

2   A says her name.

3   B says A's name, then his own.

4   C says A's and B's names then her own, and so on round the circle back to A who ends up reeling off all the names around the circle.

Communication Skills Game

Suitability:

Group size: Medium / Large

Procedure

1 Everyone has a partner.

2 Each pair then talks about what they did last night, whispering and standing close.

3 Then they talk about their favourite foods with one person standing and the other sitting down.

4 Finally they talk about the last film they saw, shouting across the room.

5 Get into groups and discuss the appropriateness of each method of communication, how they felt, etc.

Comments

★ A mix of disabilities should be included in each partnership so that points 2, 3 and 4 remain possible.

Getting to Know You

Group size: Medium / Large

Procedure

1 The whole group is spread around the room.

2 At a given signal the players must move around and shake hands with as many people as possible.

3 With every handshake they introduce themselves.

Variations

★ Give the group a time limit of one minute to shake hands with everyone in the room.

Comments

★ To make the game more accessible to those with joint problems or limited arm movement the option of nodding instead of shaking hands can be included.

★ This game gets people moving about, and means they have to acknowledge the other group members.

★ This is a good game for a group of mixed mobility, as the more mobile players will reduce the need for the less mobile to move great distances in order to shake hands.

Human Treasure Hunt

Group size: Medium / Large

Procedure

1   The leader calls out a group size and a characteristic of the people in that group and the group forms appropriately. For instance, the leader may shout:

   ★ Form into a group of four people who are the same age.

   ★ Form into a group of three people who can sing an Abba song.

   ★ Find another person with the same hero or heroine as you.

   ★ Form a group of four people who know the word for 'thank you' in a foreign language.

   ★ Form a group of three people who hate Jason Donovan and one who likes him.

   ★ Form a group of two people who watched *Neighbours* yesterday.

   ★ Find someone who hates spinach.

I am a Shoe

Group size: Small / Medium

Procedure

1   Each player looks around the room and chooses an object.

2   The leader gives everyone time to think what it would be like to be that object.

3   Players should identify three qualities that their object possesses, for example, a shoe might be warm, soft and comfortable.

4   Players then go around the room introducing themselves as their chosen object that way and shaking hands, for example: 'I am a shoe: I am warm, soft and comfortable.'

5   After a given time, players sit down and think briefly about whether the objects' qualities describe them.

6   Players should now give the object their own names and walk around introducing themselves, for example: 'I am Susan, I am warm, soft and comfortable.'

7   Afterwards, that group forms a circle and discusses the experience, doing a round of 'I felt...', or 'I discovered...'

Variations

★   Each player writes a story as if s/he were the object, or tells one aloud. Players pair off and discuss the qualities they chose in relation to themselves and their partners.

Introduction Game

Group size: Small / Medium / Large

Procedure

1. The group forms a circle and in turn each player says his/her name and another piece of information (can be silly).

2. One person says his/her own name and piece of information followed by the name and information of another player. For example: 'Ben, collects stamps; Shirish, has two brothers.'

3. The second person then says his/her name and information and those of another, continuing until everyone in circle is more familiar with names.

4. Anyone who fails to name a person correctly or forgets the piece of information drops out.

Listen

Group size: Medium

Procedure

1   The leader splits the group into pairs.

2   Let the one person in each pair talk and introduce him- or herself for 5 minutes and then change over and let the other person talk.

3   Then bring everyone back into the group. Everyone must introduce his/her partner (the leader should not warn the group that they'll be doing this beforehand).

Comments

★   A good game to demonstrate listening skills.

Name Game

Suitability:

Group size: Small / Medium

Procedure

1   The players form a circle and call out their names one by one.

2   One player is chosen to stand in the middle, and s/he calls out somebody else's name three times, as fast as s/he can.

3   The person whose name is being called has to respond by saying the central person's name before his/her own name has been called three times.

4   If the central person succeeds, the players swap places.

Names

Group size: Medium / Large

Procedure

1   The group sits in a circle.

2   Starting with the leader, each person must introduce him- or herself with a descriptive word of the same initial letter as his/her name, e.g. Exciting Emma, Super Sam.

3   When everyone has introduced themselves, the leader re-introduces him- or herself. The next person does likewise, but then repeats the leaders' introduction. The next person introduces him- or herself, the previous player and the leader. This continues around the circle.

Parent Cocktail Party

Group size: Small / Medium

Procedure

1   All the players are told to become one of their parents and pretend to be at a cocktail party.

2   Everyone moves around the room, talking to the other players they meet about your child (or children).

3   Be sure that all players talk to many different people and listen to them as well.

4   Players return to the circle and discuss what they may have learned from this about themselves, their parents or other people in the group.

Variations

★   Sit the group in a circle and ask each player to make a statement in the parental persona in turn.

★   Halfway through, ask players to switch and be their other parent.

★   Ask players to be a favourite teacher, then a much-disliked teacher.

Comments

★   Rather than insisting on people taking on the persona of a parent, it may be more appropriate to offer them a choice – parent, partner, older relative etc.

Sharing

Group size: Small / Medium / Large

Procedure

1   The leader asks each player to give his/her name and tell something new and good that has happened during the last week/day.

Variations

★ Ask the group to give their names and something exciting about the past, present or future.

★ Ask players to name a talent they have.

★ Ask everyone to say how they are feeling.

Sherlock Holmes

Group size: Small / Medium / Large

Procedure

1 Split the group into pairs.

2 In each pair, one person takes six items from their handbag or pocket and shows them to his/her partner without talking.

3 The partner does the same.

4 Each partner writes down deductions they can make about the other.

5 Bring the group back together so that everyone can share their findings. The partners should comment on the accuracy of the deductions.

Comments

★ This is a good game for starting a discussion on stereotyping.

★ If there are blind players ensure that partners name all their belongings clearly including during the feedback.

The Toilet Paper Game

Group size: Medium

Materials

Enough rolls of toilet paper for one per group.

Procedure

1   The leader splits the group into smaller groups of about 10.

2   Each group is given a roll of toilet paper and the leader asks each player to take as many or as few squares s/he chooses.

3   The leader then tells the group that s/he wants everyone to say something about themselves for every square they have (that'll get the greedy ones!).

Limited sight

See also:

Adverb Game

Suitability:

Group size: Small / Medium

Procedure

1   One player (the guesser) leaves the room, the others choose an adverb, e.g. 'slowly'.

2   When he returns s/he must find out what the adverb is by asking people to do things 'that way', e.g. 'shake hands that way' (so they would shake hands very slowly).

3   If you don't want to, or can't do what you are asked, you say 'I don't want to' (very slowly).

4   After each command the guesser must guess the word.

5   S/he can continue until s/he gets it right or gives up.

Variations

★ Leader calls out adverbs, e.g. 'nervously', and everyone moves around the room that way. (This is good as a follow-up activity, or as a means of moving into an active game or drama. It can also be used to introduce examples of adverbs if this is necessary.)

Comments

★ The guesser, when asking people to do things 'that way', should be encouraged to use actions the rest of the group are able to perform. Asking people to skip when the majority are wheelchair users does not lead anyone to a quick discovery of the adverb!

Agree / Disagree

Group size: Medium / Large

Procedure

1 The group leader decides on a set of statements. Examples could be:

   ★ boys are less tidy than girls

   ★ school is great

   ★ I eat anything

   ★ I never watch T.V.

   ★ I want everyone to be my friend

   ★ I avoid making decisions

   ★ I'm 100 per cent happy

   ★ I never argue

   ★ all old people play bingo.

2 One side of the room is for people who agree, the other for those who disagree. The space in between these forms a 'scale' of degrees of opinion.

3 Each person then moves somewhere along the scale according to their opinion or practice.

4 This 'declaration' can be used for discussion. As in other games, no criticism is to be made of anyone's choice.

Variations

   ★ Each person chooses where s/he would *like* to be, not necessarily where s/he would be in reality.

   ★ Each person explains why s/he is choosing a particular point.

★ Split room into two and have a dialogue between the two sides on 'why *we* are right!'

Comments

★ The leader must decide how controversial to make the statements.

Alphabet Game

Suitability:

Group size: Medium / Large

Procedure

1   Ask the group to line up in alphabetic order according to surname.

2   Once this has been done, ask them to line up alphabetically by home towns.

3   Now ask them to line up chronologically, according to date of birth.

Variation

★ Continue with as many facts that can be ordered as you wish.

Comments

★ Provide chairs occasionally along the line for those unable to stand for long. If there are no wheelchair users, you could arrange a line of chairs.

★ If there are players unable to stand for long or with mobility problems, keep the group small.

Animal Noises

Group size: Medium

Procedure

1 Players stand in a circle, with one person blindfolded and standing in the middle.

2 The leader guides the blindfolded person to someone in the circle.

3 The blindfolded person says the name of an animal and the player s/he is standing by has to imitate the sound of the animal.

4 The blindfolded person must identify who the person is.

5 If the blindfolded player does not guess immediately, s/he should continue to ask the other players to make animal noises.

6 When the blindfolded person has guessed, the imitator becomes the blind-folded player.

Comments

★ Do not choose a hearing-impaired person to be blindfolded.

Beautiful Things

Group size: Small / Medium / Large

Procedure

1   A leader is chosen who tells the other players that s/he will describe something that they think of as very beautiful, nice or good. S/he must not name it at any point.

2   S/he describes the object that s/he is thinking of as fully as possible, but in unfavourable terms: in other words, s/he must try to make it sound like something that isn't beautiful, nice or good, even though it is. For example, the leader might choose 'flower', normally considered beautiful. In order to make it sound ugly, s/he might say: 'It doesn't last very long. If you touch it, it may fall apart. It usually has bugs on it, and after a while it starts to smell bad.' Describing a pizza, s/he might say: 'It's very messy most of the time. It's too spicy. If it's hot it burns you. It has all kinds of stuff on top of it. You won't like it cold.'

3   After s/he has described the object, the players are given five chances to guess it.

4   Whoever guesses correctly becomes the new leader.

Data Processing

Suitability:

Group size: Small / Medium / Large

Procedure

1   The leader calls out a category and the group must order themselves in a line accordingly. Examples could be:

      first names, alphabetically,

      birthdays, chronologically

      favourite ice-cream flavours,

      Zodiac signs (lead into game for 12 groups).

Comments

★ If there are a large number of players with walking difficulties keep the line length/group size small.

★ This is a good way to split a large group up into smaller numbers, and promotes mixing.

Down on the Farm

Suitability:

Group size: Medium / Large

Procedure

1   The leader goes round whispering to all the people in the group the name of an animal. Make sure there are 2 cows, 2 frogs etc. but only 1 duck!

2   Everyone has to make a noise and/or an action imitating their animal until they find their partners.

Variations

★ If you are using this as a blind awareness game, only allow players to make the noise of their animals and make sure they keep their eyes shut when finding their partners. But don't play this with wheelchair users or deaf players.

Find the Same

Suitability:

Group size: Small

Procedure

1   Everyone must close their eyes.

2   By feel, players have to find another player who has something in common with themselves. For example, someone else wearing jeans or trainers, or with short hair.

Comments

★ This game should only be played in situations where the group knows the members well. It may not be suitable in mixed groups.

★ Not suitable for wheelchair users because of safety.

★ A good game for promoting blind awareness.

Gibberish

Suitability:

Group size: Small

Procedure

1   The leader splits the group into pairs and suggests the subject of a conversation they must hold.

2   The leader then explains that no recognisable words may be used.

3   Each pair will talk in 'gibberish', making up words and sounds. The idea is to develop in intensity of expression excluding real words.

4   Ideas for conversation:

lend me some money;

where were you last night?

go home, your house has been burgled;

it was the funniest game I've ever seen;

did you see that TV programme last night?

Variations

★   Instead of sounds, or made-up words, numbers can be used.

Ha Ha Ha!

Suitability:

Group size: Medium

Procedure

1 Everyone sits in a circle and holds hands with the people on either side of them.

2 The leader squeezes the hand of the person on his/her left.

3 People pass on the squeeze until it reaches the person at the end of the circle, to the right of the leader.

4 The person to the right of the leader now yells 'ha'.

5 The person to his right yells 'ha, ha'.

6 The person to his right yells 'ha, ha, ha', and so on until the laughs reach the leader.

7 Continue until it breaks up.

Variations

★ Try completing a circle of squeezes and then laughs as fast as possible.

★ On the second round, start the squeezes and laughs off simultaneously so both are going round at the same time: this adds to the confusion!

Hole in the Bucket

Group size: Medium / Large

Materials

4 buckets, 2 plastic cups.

Procedure

1 The leader splits the group into 2 teams and makes them form a line.

2 A bucket is placed at the front and at the back of each line. The 2 buckets at the front are filled with water.

3 Using a plastic cup, the teams have to fill the bucket at the back by passing the cup from hand to hand.

4 After five minutes the leader should stop them – the team which has transported the most water wins.

Variations

★ To increase the difficulty, try using plastic plates instead of cups.

★ To increase the soaking of the team members, use a cup with holes in it!

Comments

★ Try to even out the types of disability within each team so the chances remain fair.

I'll Bet You Can't

Group size: Medium

Procedure

1   One player is chosen as a leader.

2   The leader tells the group something s/he would like to do, for example, 'I would like to build a wagon'.

3   A player then challenges the leader by naming two things that s/he does not think could be used to do it, for example, 'I bet you can't use a pillow or a hamburger to build a wagon'.

4   The leader must give a reasonable way that s/he could use one of the two things named to do what s/he'd like to do. For instance: 'I could use the pillow to make a comfortable seat in my wagon.'

5   The leader keeps the lead as long as s/he can think of a way to use one of the objects named to do the chosen job.

6   When the leader gets stuck, the player whose suggestion caught him/her out becomes the new leader.

Make a Story

Group size: Medium

Procedure

1   The group should sit in a circle.

2   The leader starts a story, then stops and the next person takes over.

3   Carry on until the last person in the circle, who finishes the story.

Variations

★   Each player stops mid-sentence.

★   The person speaking chooses who carries on the story next.

The Ordering Game

Group size: Medium

Materials

Nine cards with each of the following words and its opposite printed on:

Card 1 – cold/hot

Card 2 – dull/bright

Card 3 – hard/soft

Card 4 – loud/quiet

Card 5 – wet/dry

Card 6 – light/heavy

Card 7 – small/large

Card 8 – dark/light

Card 9 – rough/smooth.

Procedure

1   The players form a line, and the cards are placed in a pile on a table.

2   The first player in line takes the top card, for example, Card 1, cold/hot.

3   S/he then tells the other players to put themselves in that order, e.g:
    'Name things going from cold to hot.'

4   The next player in line must name something very cold; the next,
    something not quite so cold; the next, something even less cold; the next,
    something warmer; and the last, something very hot. So, in a group of
    five people, the whole line might be: ice, milk, tap water, cup of coffee,
    the sun.

5   If a player makes a mistake, the next player must correctly name
    something for that place.

6   When the whole group has contributed a word to the line, the first player moves to the end of the line, the second player chooses a new card and the game continues.

7   A player gets one point for each correct answer and is responsible for keeping his/her own score.

8   After five cards have been used, the player with the most points wins.

9   If the game is tied, players may wish to draw one or more additional cards to determine a winner.

Partner Conversations

Suitability:

Group size: Small / Large

Procedure

1   Divide the group into partners.

2   Ask them to hold hands or put their arms around each other.

3   Each pair must find another pair and hold a conversation with them. Partners alternate in speaking one word, until a sentence is formed. (It becomes an exercise in mind-reading.)

4   Once one pair has formed a sentence, the other pair responds.

Variations

★   Use teams of 3 or 4 instead of pairs.

★   Move pairs on after a given time.

Pass Squeeze

Group size: Medium / Large

Procedure

1   Everyone sits in a circle holding hands.

2   The leader starts by squeezing the hand of the person on his or her right who must then pass the squeeze on.

3   This continues round the circle.

4   After speed it up and add a sound too, such as: 'oooh'

5   Now send the squeeze in the opposite direction with another sound like: 'aaaagh!'

6   Then try and get more than one squeeze and sound going round the circle in different directions at the same time.

Comments

★   If playing this game with deaf players omit the noises.

Speechless

Group size: Medium

Procedure

1 One player is chosen as a leader and stands before the rest of the group.

2 Players ask the leader questions and indicate one word that cannot be included in the answer. They should try to stump the leader by choosing words that usually would be used to answer their questions. For example, a player might ask: 'What class are you in? And don't use the word 4'.

3 The leader has to answer each question truthfully, without using the prohibited word. For example, to 'What class are you in? And don't use the word 4', s/he might answer, 'I'm in the class that comes after Class 3'.

4 The leader maintains his/her lead until asked a question that s/he cannot answer.

5 The player who caught out the leader then takes his or her place.

Comments

★ This game is more effective if the players know each other fairly well.

Tick Tock

Suitability:

Group size: Small / Medium

Materials

Pen or similar small item.

Procedure

1   The leader has a pen or similar item.

2   S/he passes it to the right and says 'This is a tick'.

3   Player 1 says 'a what?'. The leader replies, 'a tick'.

4   Player 1 passes it to Player 2 and says, 'this is a tick'. Player 2: 'a what?'. Player 1: 'a what?'. Leader: 'a tick'. Player 1: 'a tick'. Player 2: 'this is a tick'.

5   Player 2 then passes on the pen, and the game continues.

6   At the end, either begin again with the pen going to the left, 'a tock', or pass two around in opposite directions. Try to return both to the leader.

Water Pirates

Group size: Medium

Materials

Clothes, water pistol.

Procedure

1   A pirate is blindfolded, half-a-dozen clothes tucked into his/her belt/wheelchair and given a water-pistol as a weapon.

2   Everyone else has to sneak up and steal a piece of clothing without getting squirted.

Comments

★ Roles can be adapted according to the disability, e.g. while a blind person can be the pirate, a deaf person cannot.

Who Am I?

Group size: Medium / Large

Procedure

1   Each person chooses to become a famous character, perhaps from history, entertainment, literature or politics.

2   The leader asks each person to sit separately and concentrate on:

> the kind of personality the character has
>
> their mannerisms
>
> the way they talk
>
> what they say.

3   When everyone is ready they act as the character they have chosen and move around to introduce themselves to each other.

4   They can also hold conversations with one another making sure they retain all the characteristics of the famous person.

Word Tickle

Group size: Small

Procedure

1   The group is divided into pairs.

2   One person says as many nice things about the other as s/he can think of – tickling with words.

3   Change over after two minutes.

Zoom Eeek

Suitability:

Group size: Medium

Procedure

1   The group forms a circle.

2   Everyone practises making the noises 'Zoom' – the sound of a racing car – and 'Eeek' – the screech of brakes. Add actions to go with them.

3   The first person says 'Zoom' turning to the left or right. This is the direction the imaginary car is going, so the person turned to carries on the 'Zoom'.

4   Go round the circle once with everyone saying 'Zoom'.

5   Now the players have the choice of saying 'Zoom' or 'Eeek'. If someone says 'Eeek' the car has screeched to a halt and goes back the same way it came.

Comments

★   Play fast for true fun!

Limited hearing

see also:

Balloon

Group size: Small / Medium

Procedure

1 Sit the group in a circle, one player standing in the centre with a balloon.

2 Number everyone.

3 The centre player holds the balloon up, calls out a number and lets it fall.

4 The player of that number must catch the balloon before it falls to the ground.

5 If s/he fails, that player takes over the centre.

Comments

★ This game can be played with larger groups, subdivided into smaller circles.

★ When playing with those less mobile or dextrous, the groups and circle should be kept small.

★ If points are going to be awarded the groups should be of a similar ability level, e.g. a group of those who are most mobile, a group of people with little arm movement etc.

Contact

Suitability:

Group size: Medium

Procedure

1   One person leaves the room.

2   The remaining players sit in a circle and hold hands.

3   A player is chosen to send a message around the circle by squeezing his/her neighbour's hand.

4   The squeeze message is repeated by each player until it gets back to the sender.

5   The player comes back from outside and the aim is for him/her to guess the squeeze message by 'feeling' it.

Do I Bark?

Group size: Small / Medium

Materials

Sticky labels.

Procedure

1 Names of animals are written on sticky labels.

2 Somebody is chosen and one label is stuck to his/her back. The player must not see what is written on it.

3 The player is allowed to ask each of the other people one question in an attempt to find out what kind of an animal s/he is supposed to be. Questions could be, 'Am I brown?', 'Have I got thick fur?', 'Do I bark?'. The questions can only be those which require a response 'yes' or 'no'.

4 As soon as the player thinks s/he knows s/he can ask: 'Am I a –?'

5 If the guess is correct, a new person is chosen.

6 The winner is the person who guesses what s/he is in the least number of questions.

Electricity Current Game

Group size: Medium / Large

Procedure

1   The group should stand in a circle holding hands. A volunteer stands in the middle.

2   The leader explains that the players are an electricity grid. An electrical current will be passed through them. Each player must pass it on to the next by squeezing hands.

3   Two to four people are chosen to say 'ping' when the current goes through them.

4   'Pingers' can change the direction of the current by squeezing the hand of the person who just passed on the pulse.

5   When the player in the centre of the circle spots the current – the hands squeezing – s/he swaps places with the player who has been caught.

Comments

★   The current does not always have to move, and can be passed on at different paces, more quickly or more slowly.

Fear in a Hat

Suitability:

Group size: Medium

Procedure

1   The players are arranged in a circle.

2   Everyone, including the leader, must complete this sentence (anonymously): 'In this class [or group, or whatever] I am afraid that –' Put the scraps of paper in the hat in the centre.

3   Pass the hat around the circle.

4   Each player must pull one piece of paper out and read it, enlarge on the sentence and try to express what the person was feeling. For example, the leader should read the first one, and might say: 'In this class I am afraid that I will be laughed at–[continues talking] I am afraid to say my feelings because everyone laughs at me, so I never say anything.'

5   Continue round the circle.

6   The leader must make sure that everyone just listens, and does not comment. No arguing or comment is allowed.

7   Then discuss what was noticed or discovered.

Variations

★   Instead of fear in a hat, put in worries, gripes or wishes.

★   Use two hats and explore likes and dislikes in a hat.

Finder's Clap

Suitability:

Group size: Medium / Large

Procedure

1   A volunteer ('finder') leaves the room and an object is hidden.

2   The 'finder' comes back. The group clap louder and louder as the 'finder' nears the object.

3   Once the object is found, another person is chosen to become the 'finder'.

Comments

★   When playing this with a group including deaf people, stamp feet. The vibration will indicate how close the 'finder' is, but remember that foot stamping excludes those players in wheelchairs or with leg weakness.

Goods Wagon Relay

Group size: Medium / Large

Procedure

1   The group is lined up in teams of about 10.

2   The first person in each team is the train and runs down the room to a line, returns backwards and picks up the second player (a wagon).

3   Both run forward to the line, shunt backwards and pick up a third.

4   This continues until all the wagons have been picked up. The first complete train wins.

Comments

★ Only adept wheelchair users can be included.

★ It may be safer for wheelchair users to make up one team.

★ If playing with people with mobility difficulties the distance to the line should be short.

Human Structures

Group size: Small / Medium / Large

Procedure

1   The leader splits the group into smaller groups of between 2 and 8 people.

2   Each group constructs a particular structure by linking themselves together. For example:

   a suspension bridge

   an arched bridge

   a tree

   a crane

   a modern building

   an aeroplane/helicopter

   a car/truck/bus

   a ship

   a tower

   a dome

   a temple

   a cathedral.

Variations

★ Once the structure is made the players should try to move around without falling.

Comments

★ Groups containing a mixture of disabilities will be more effective.

Leader of the Orchestra

Suitability:

Group size: Large / Medium

Procedure

1   The players sit in a circle.

2   One person is chosen to leave the room.

3   While s/he is out, one player in the circle is nominated as leader of the orchestra. S/he begins to play any instrument in mime, and all others in the circle must imitate and mime the same instrument.

4   When everyone is performing, the player is called in from outside and into the middle of the circle.

5   The leader of the orchestra then begins changing instruments from time to time, and the rest of the circle must follow. They should follow the leader without appearing to watch him/her.

6   The player in the middle must try to find out who is the leader of the orchestra.

Comments

★   Players with little arm movement should be chosen as the leader or guesser.

Matchbox Merriment

Group size: Medium / Large

Materials

Matchbox covers.

Procedure

1   The group is split into two teams and each team is given a matchbox cover.

2   The first member of each team puts the matchbox on his/her nose and, without anyone using their hands, the box must be passed from nose to nose until it reaches the end of the team.

3   If the matchbox is dropped the team has to start again.

4   The first team to get the matchbox to the end is the winner.

Comments

★ A similar mix of disabilities should be included in each team.

★ Ensure that a player with little movement is placed between players with extensive movement.

Mill and Grab

Group size: Medium / Large

Procedure

1   Everyone should mill around the room.

2   The leader calls a number, e.g. '5'.

3   Members make circles of 5 and hold hands.

4   Anyone left over goes to the middle of the room where it may be possible to form another group.

5   The leader must wait until all the groups are ready, and then call another number. If the leader wants groups of 7 for the next game, s/he stops with 7, tells groups to keep their 7 and sit down.

6   Emphasise that groups must be mixed, boys and girls, teachers and pupils, etc.

Variations

★ The players close their eyes (not suitable for deaf players but a good blind awareness game).

★ The players play in silence (not suitable for blind players but a good deaf awareness game).

★ Play the game in slow motion.

★ Play as noisily as possible.

★ Choose an adverb, e.g. childishly, and play in the manner of the adverb.

Comments

★ Variations must be carefully selected according to the variety of disabilities contained within the group. Playing in silence may make it very difficult for blind people to join in.

★ This can be a good game for raising awareness of visual or auditory impairments.

Pack of Cards

Suitability:

Group size: Medium / Large

Materials

One pack of cards with the jokers removed.

Procedure

1   Before the group arrives the leader must hide all the cards in various places around the room. Put them at a variety of heights so they can be seen by and are accessible to all players.

2   Split the group into four teams and name them – Hearts, Diamonds, Spades and Clubs.

3   On the word 'GO' each team has to search the room for cards from their suit.

4   If people find a card that is not in their suit they must leave it where it is.

5   The first team to collect a complete suit wins.

Variations

★   Give a time limit: the team with the most cards wins.

Paper Fish

Suitability:

Group size: Medium

Materials

A paper cut-out fish, a plate and a rolled-up newspaper for each player.

Procedure

1   All the plates are lined up on the floor at one end of the room.

2   The players stand at the opposite end and are each given a fish and a newspaper.

3   The players must waft their fishes along the floor onto the plates, using the newspaper.

4   The first fish wafted onto a plate wins.

Comments

★   If some players have difficulties bending down, or are wheelchair users with limited upper body movement, play the game along a long table. Straws can be used to blow the fishes along the table if this is easier.

Sign Game

Suitability:

Group size: Medium

Procedure

1   The players form a circle and each one adopts a sign, such as a raised hand, a nod of the head or a twitch.

2   One by one each player performs his or her sign for the group.

3   Then, one player makes his or her own sign followed by that of someone else.

4   That person then makes his or her own sign followed by that of someone else, and so on.

Comments

★   It must be remembered that players with limited movement may only be able to perform some of the signs.

Silent Island

Suitability:

Group size: Small

Materials

A lump of clay large enough for each group of 7 people to gather around a table and work together. Clay should be of the malleable, non-drying variety; also leaves, twigs and toothpicks or sticks should be provided.

Procedure

1 A group of 5 to 7 players gathers around a table with the clay in the centre. Without speaking to each other, the group should push and knead the clay into a mass. Then the group must make the lump into an island, adding castles, caves, mountains, rivers etc.

2 Still without talking, each player must mark a boundary for his or her own area and build a shelter or home, using any other materials he or she wishes.

3 The leader asks the group to hold an island council meeting. At this meeting, players must elect a leader and make whatever decisions are needed for survival or interaction on the island.

4 At this point the group can stop and discuss what and why they decided and what problem they encountered, or go further (see variations).

Variations

★ Continue improvising incidents of island life.

★ Use a large piece of paper and chalk instead of clay.

Spirals

Group size: Medium

Procedure

1 One person stands in the middle of the room.

2 Everyone else links hands in a long chain and coils round the central person, forming a spiral.

3 When the spiral is complete, the central person must duck down and crawl through legs, still holding hands and leading the line behind him or her, to undo the spiral.

Comments

★ If the central player is unable to duck down, he or she can wait until the coil is formed and then yell 'snap', at which the coil must quickly unwind of its own accord.

Tails

Suitability:

Group size: Medium

Materials

String.

Procedure

1 All players are given a length of string which they loosely attach to the back of their trousers or waistbands. The string should be of sufficient length to drag along the floor.

2 On the signal to start, players try to tread on other players' tails so as to detach them from the waistband while keeping their own tails intact. Any amount of dodging is allowed.

3 The last player left with a tail is the winner.

Comments

★ Not really suitable for wheelchair users unless the group consists of all wheelchair users and tails are yanked from the back of players' wheelchairs.

Waterchild

Group size: Medium

Materials

Paper cups.

Procedure

1 The group stands or sits in circles of about 10.

2 Each player puts an empty paper cup between his/her teeth.

3 One cup is filled with water.

4 The aim is to pour the water into the next cup without players using their hands.

5 The team with the most water in the last cup is the winner.

Comments

★ Groups must be structured carefully so a mobile player is placed next to a less mobile player to compensate for movement difficulties.

★ Wheelchair users should only be placed next to each other if at least one has good upper body movement.

Winking Murder

Suitability:

Group size: Medium / Large

Procedure

1 A volunteer goes out of the room and the remaining players sit in a circle with their eyes closed.

2 The leader (who is not taking part) chooses a murderer by tapping a player on the head.

3 The volunteer comes back in and stands in the centre of the circle.

4 The murderer has to wink at others and then they must die as dramatically as possible. They must not, however, stare at the murderer and give him/her away.

5 The volunteer in the middle must find the murderer as quickly as possible. Then it becomes the murderer's turn to leave the room.

Woolly Fun

Suitability:

Group size: Medium / Large

Materials

Pieces of wool varying in length.

Procedure

1 The leader hides all the pieces of wool around the room.

2 Everyone must search around for the pieces of wool. The winner is not the player with the most pieces of wool but the one whose wool will make the longest line with the pieces laid end to end.

3 When all the wool has been found, or after a set time, each player lays out their pieces of wool until the winner is found!

Comments

★ Ensure all the pieces of wool are at an accessible height to all players.

Limited mobility

see also:

Air-Raid Shelter

Group size: Small / Medium

Procedure

1 Divide into groups of 8–10.

2 Each group member should adopt a specific role, different disability, a stereotype or an occupation, e.g. a doctor, an athlete, a teacher, movie-star, mother, housewife (these can be picked out from a hat).

3 The leader should tell the groups that they are in an air-raid shelter after an atom bomb has fallen. The shelter is only big enough and with enough air and food for six people, therefore each group must get rid of several members.

4 Each group member must argue as to why s/he should be allowed to survive.

5 A group decision must be reached as to who goes and stays: no suicides or murders allowed.

6 Set a time limit for the decision.

7 Later, discuss how the group interacted during the process of making the decision, whether each person played an active or passive role, how satisfied each was with his/her role, etc.

Variations

★ Instead of an air-raid shelter, use a life raft or desert island or space ship as the scenario.

Animal Happy Families

Group size: Medium / Large

Materials

Paper.

Procedure

1 Names of animals are written on strips of paper and handed to players as they enter the room.

2 When music stops/hand is waved, make noise or action of animal.

3 Sit down in groups after finding the same animals.

Comments

★ This is a good way to sort people into groups or pairs and encourage mixing.

★ It must be emphasised at the beginning that players can make the noise of the animal, perform an action, or do both.

★ If some players are blind or cannot read, the names of the animals could be written in Braille, or the leader could tell each person his/her animal as s/he enters the room.

Arch Game

Suitability:

Group size: Medium

Procedure

1 Two players raise their hands and form an arch.

2 The others make a chain and walk through the arch singing a phrase, e.g. 'school is the best, school is the best… one, two, three'. Whatever phrase is chosen it must end in 'one, two, three'.

3 The pair forming the arch lower and raise their arms on the words 'one, two, three'.

4 On the third time the arch is left down and the player trapped in it is out.

5 When a second person is 'caught' the two 'caught' players form the new arch and the game restarts.

Famous People

Suitability:

Group size: Medium / Large

Materials

Sticky labels.

Procedure

1   Write famous names on sticky labels.

2   Stick one to each person's back.

3   Players must move around the group asking questions (eliciting only yes/no answers) and try to guess who they are.

4   As each player discovers who they are, they should stick their labels to their fronts and continue to help others.

Variations

★ For younger players use characters from nursery rhymes or fairytales.

★ You could use the names of famous couples, for example Romeo and Juliet, Tom and Jerry. Once the players have guessed their own names, they must find their partners by asking similar questions requiring yes/no answers.

★ Labels need to be stuck to the back of the players' wheelchairs where applicable.

Farmyard Fun

Suitability:

Group size: Medium / Large

Materials

Paper, pencils.

Procedure

1   One person acts as judge and whispers the name of a farm animal to each person in the room.

2   On the signal 'Go' everyone has to imitate the animal, making noises and/or performing an action.

3   After a few minutes the judge stops the group and hands out a piece of paper and pencil to each player.

4   Each player has to write down all the animal noises they heard.

5   The person with the most correct answers is the winner.

Comments

★   Spare people should be available to take dictation from those unable to write.

Group Outing

Group size: Large / Small / Medium

Procedure

1   The group sits in a circle.

2   The leader starts – 'Last Sunday I went to the seaside and took with me – a jar of pickled parsnips'.

3   The next person repeats what the leader has said and adds an object.

4   This continues around a circle. Those not able to remember the story drop out.

Gripes Auction

Group size: Medium / Large

Materials

A card or piece of paper for each person and pencils.

Procedure

1   The leader holds a series of cards, each containing a gripe:

Little children	Dogs	Drama Lessons
Babysitting	The weather	Smokers
Pocket money	Students	Dentists
Films on TV	School meals	Violence
Newspapers	Sports	Sexism
Parents	Cats	Oppression
School	Homework	Police people
Brothers	Books	Fashions
Sisters	Teachers	Shopping
Youth Club	Grandparents	Vandalism
Holidays	Pollution	Doctors
Facilities for young people (recreation)	Gossip	

2   All the gripes are read out first and then each gripe is put up for auction.

3   Each person has 100 points to spend and cannot bid over this.

4   When the auction is over the people who have cards explain why their particular gripe is important and how it affects their lives.

Variations

★   Brainstorm your own list of gripes before playing.

Identifi-Picture

Suitability:

Group size: Medium

Procedure

1 A player is chosen to stand with his/her back to the rest of the group.

2 Another player describes someone in the room and the player with her/his back turned must guess who is being described.

3 When the player with her/his back turned guesses correctly s/he chooses someone to stand at the front and someone to describe.

4 Discuss how people described others; what seemed to be the important cues.

It's a Verbal Knockout

Suitability:

Group size: Small / Medium / Large

Procedure

1   A pair are chosen and they sit facing each other in the centre of the group.

2   The pair have to challenge each other verbally for thirty seconds, from a chosen category:

Chatterbox – both persons must keep up a continuous stream of talk simultaneously.

Nonsense – both persons are given an emotion to express (e.g. fear, joy). These must be expressed with nonsense sounds simultaneously.

Show-off – in turn, each must try to be 'one-up' on the other person with fictional facts about themselves.

3   At the end of thirty seconds, the group decides who won the round.

4   Another person then challenges the winner.

Knee Tag

Suitability:

Group size: Medium

Procedure

1   Players must go round the room and touch knee to knee with every person, saying 'Hi, I'm – and this is my knee'.

Variations

★ If a player meets the same person again s/he must select another part of his/her body to introduce to him/her.

★ Place a time limit on the knee tag.

Comments

★ Use other parts of the body if they are more suitable for those taking part.

★ A good game for mixed abilities because those able to move their bodies will touch with those who cannot, therefore all can participate.

Mime Rhyme

Suitability:

Group size: Medium

Procedure

1   One player is chosen to stand in the middle of the room.

2   S/he tells the rest of the group 'I'm thinking of a word that rhymes with …'.

3   The rest of the players must try to work out what the word is, but they can't say what their guess is, they have to mime it. So for a word that rhymes with 'deep', players might rest their head on their hands for 'sleep' or wipe away tears for 'weep'.

4   The player in the middle of the room must respond to the mimes by saying 'No, it's not "sleep"', 'No it's not "weep"' and the players have to carry on miming they have successfully guessed the word and communicated this to the person in the middle.

5   The player who mimes the correct word goes to the middle of the room and the game begins again.

Mime the Lie

Group size: Small / Medium

Procedure

1   The players form a circle.

2   One player is chosen to start miming an action, e.g. painting a wall, and the person to the right asks the question: 'What are you doing?'

3   The person doing the action has to lie, so maybe they would reply 'tap dancing'.

4   The questioner then has to mime tap dancing, and the player to his/her right asks what s/he is doing, and so on.

Comments

★   How suitable this game is for the people playing depends on their level of awareness. When people are next to someone with a disability they must think of a suitable action for them to mime. It can lead onto discussion of how people felt, what they discovered, where their knowledge is lacking etc.

★   This is a good game for raising awareness of disabilities.

Musical Hats

Group size: Medium

Materials

A selection of hats – one less than the number of players – and a record, cassette or CD player.

Procedure

1   The players are told to sit in a circle and are given the assortment of hats.

2   The leader switches on the record player, and the players start to pass around the hats.

3   When the music stops any player without a hat on drops out.

4   Sufficient hats are taken away so that again there is one less hat than the number of players, and the music begins again.

5   The last player left is the winner.

Rainforest Morning

Group size: Small / Medium / Large

Procedure

1   Everyone sits, closes their eyes and thinks of an animal.

2   The leader tells the group to pretend that dawn is coming and the animals are beginning to wake up. Softly at first, everyone makes the sound of their animals and does an appropriate action; gradually increasing the noise until it has become a morning chorus.

3   The leader tells the animals to stretch as they awake, and after they are awake, to start moving around the rainforest greeting other animals.

Comments

★ Offer players the choice of making a noise, performing an action or doing both depending on ability.

Sharing Circle

Group size: Small / Medium / Large

Procedure

1   The players sit in a circle and take turns saying the name of the person to their left and something they like about that person.

Comments

★ If there are blind people within the group it would be useful initially for each player in turn to introduce him- or herself, so that the blind members of the group know everyone's positions.

What is my Job?

Group size: Small / Medium / Large

Procedure

1   Each player writes the name of an occupation or job on a piece of paper and five words that are closely related to that job, e.g. dentist – tooth, drill, filling, mouth, gums. These are the words the 'occupation' person cannot use when s/he helps the players to guess his/her job. Players should try to choose words that will make it difficult for the 'occupation' player to succeed.

2   The pieces of paper are gathered up, shuffled, and re-distributed.

3   The 'occupation' person faces the group and describes his/her occupation without saying the words written on the piece of paper. Someone should be appointed to check this.

3   When another player guesses the occupation, s/he becomes the 'occupation' person.

What's the Rule?

Group size: Medium

Procedure

1   The group forms a circle.

2   One person goes out – the questioner.

3   Others choose a rule, e.g. 'female players tell lies/male players tell the truth'; 'scratch your head before answering'. (A good rule to begin with is answer every question as if you were the person on your right.)

4   When the questioner comes back s/he must work out the rule by asking people questions about themselves. Players must answer questions honestly, according to the rules.

Comments

★ Rules can be hard or very simple, according to age and experience. Rules can be visual (scratch head before answering), or structural (each answer begins with the next letter of the alphabet).

★ If cards with the rules are provided then unsuitable rules won't be chosen.

★ Don't have action rules for those with limited movement, or those with sight difficulties.

The Word Wizard

Group size: Medium / Large

Materials

Pencil and paper.

Procedure:

(The leader gives the instructions below slowly, and one at a time, with pauses between.)

1. 'I am a wizard, I am taking away all your words. But as I am generous, you may have four of them back.

2. 'Decide on four words you want to keep out of all the words in the world.

3. 'Find a partner, communicate using only your four words, plus gestures.......(pause for everyone to do this).

4. 'Now you may share words with your partner, so that you have up to eight words.

5. 'Change partners and communicate with your new partner with these eight words.

6. 'Share words, so that now you have sixteen.'

7. (Repeat, changing partners four to six times.)

Variation

★ Players write the words down through the game and use their trial lists to try to write a poem.

Limited upper body strength and mobility

See also:

Animal Race

Suitability:

Group size: Medium / Large

Procedure

1   Group splits into teams of about 10.

2   Each player chooses a different animal, e.g. hen, caterpillar, crab.

3   The teams then line up for a relay race. The difference is that each player must move like their chosen animal and/or make an appropriate noise.

4   The first team back wins.

Build a Machine

Group size: Medium / Large

Procedure

1 Each player decides on a simple repetitive action and/or noise e.g. 'choo-choo', whistling, screeching, clapping.

2 Players combine in pairs, working in rhythm to make a simple machine.

3 Players should then move into groups of four (two pairs) and continue making the group bigger and bigger until the whole group is one big machine.

Variations

★ A leader nominates one person to start and chooses others to join the machine one by one.

Errrrr...

Group size: Small / Medium

Procedure

1   Only the leader is aware of the rules. S/he explains to the rest of the group that s/he has found a common feature to certain towns, and the group must guess what it is.

2   To find out, each member of the group must name a town, and the leader will say whether or not the town is one of those with the common feature.

3   The leader knows that the common feature is the way the players ask the questions. Any town prefixed by 'er' is included. So, the question 'Is, um, er, Newcastle, one of them?' the leader would reply 'yes'; to the question 'What about Cheltenham?', the reply would be 'no'.

4   As the players guess the theme, they continue to ask questions to keep the game going and to give the other players extra clues until everyone has worked it out. You know everyone has worked it out when everyone gives a town correctly.

Variations

★ Choose other rules to categorise the towns.

★ Instead of towns, use flowers, animals, countries, famous people, etc.

Farmyard

Suitability:

Group size: Medium / Large

Procedure

1   The leader divides the players into groups of four.

2   Each group chooses one member to be a dog, one to be a cow, one to be a sheep, and one to be a chicken.

3   When the leader says 'GO' all the animals wander round the room making a noise and/or an action of their animal. The aim is for the same animals to gather together.

Comments

★ This is a good way to mix groups for the next activity.

Guess Who Said It

Group size: Small / Large

Procedure

1   The players form a circle.

2   One person leaves the room.

3   Three or four people make positive statements about the absent player trying to include specialised information that not everyone might know about the person.

4   When s/he returns, s/he stands in the middle of the circle, and the statements are repeated to him/her one at a time, while s/he tries to guess who said each one.

Comments

★   The leader must insist on receiving only positive statements.

Huggy Bear

Suitability:

Group size: Medium / Large

Procedure

1   The players mingle around the room, going as fast or slow as they like.

2   The leader calls out a number, and the players must get into a group of that number and hold each other in a hug.

3   The leader then calls another number, and another.

4   The game can end with the number of the whole group being called out so that everyone has one big hug.

Comments

★   A good game for mixed abilities as those that do not have the upper body movement to hug will be hugged by those around them and therefore are included.

Islands

Group size: Medium

Materials

String/rope.

Procedure

1 Different lengths of rope or string are scattered around the floor in circles (the islands).

2 Players wander around at will. On a given command they must land on an 'island'.

3 On further instruction the players wander off again and a number of 'islands' are removed. This encourages players to share 'islands'.

4 Towards the end there will be only one 'island' left and all will have to attempt to land on it.

Comments

★ This is a great exercise in group co-operation.

★ Blind people with guiders should be able to take part.

★ Placing chairs on the islands will spare people with mobility difficulties from standing for a long time.

★ If some players are wheelchair users or have walking difficulties there should always be islands big enough to take a wheelchair or a chair.

Lawyer

Suitability:

Group size: Medium

Procedure

1 The players sit in a circle.

2 One player is chosen to be the lawyer and sits in the middle of the circle.

3 The leader says: 'Starting now, you must not answer when I speak to you, the person on your left will do so for you. You must not smile, nod your head or respond to me in any way, do you all understand?'

4 Anyone who answers is out.

5 The lawyer then proceeds to ask individuals questions. If they answer they are out.

Linked Animals

Group size: Medium

Procedure

1 The players sit or stand in a widely-spaced circle.

2 One person imitates an animal using a sound and/or an action.

3 When someone has guessed it, the next person in the circle has to imitate an animal beginning with the last letter of the previous animal. For example, after a frog, a goat; after a goat, a tadpole; and so on.

The Machine Game

Suitability:

Group size: Medium / Large

Procedure

1   The players are divided into teams of about 6.

2   The teams go to separate parts of the room.

3   Each team decides on a machine it will be. Each member decides on the part of the machine that s/he will act out. For example, if a team chooses to be a washing machine, one player could hold out his or her arms and be the tub, another could be different buttons and another could be the lid.

4   Each team practises being the machine it has chosen.

5   Each team takes a turn presenting its machine to the other teams who must guess what kind of machine it is.

Comments

★   It should be emphasised that all members of a team are to be parts of only one machine.

Machines 2

Group size: Small / Medium

Procedure

1   The leader should divide the group into smaller groups of 5 to 12 people. Each group creates a machine with moving parts.

2   The leader should see that each person in the group is involved, either as part of the machine, operating it, being a product of it, etc.

3   Each group then shows the machine to the other groups.

Variations

1   Add noises.

2   Assign a specific machine to each group, for example:

       laugh machine

       juke box

       trouble-making machine

       insult machine.

3   Make a factory, combining the machines of the whole group.

Noah's Ark

Group size: Medium / Large

Materials

Pieces of paper with the names of animals written on them, a pair of each sort of animal; and a bag.

Procedure

1   All the players take a piece of paper from a bag of animal pairs.

2   Making the noise of the animal, or miming its movements, they must find their partners.

Variations

★ Add a few unusual or made-up animals to make the game more interesting and last a bit longer.

★ Blindfold the players and allow them to make noises only if you are using this as a blind awareness game. But remember that for safety reasons wheelchair users cannot take part in this training.

Comments

★ If there are blind players remember to tell them their animal!

Quick Line-up

Suitability:

Group size: Medium / Large

Procedure

1   The group is split up into four teams standing in lines. The group forms a square, one team per side, everyone facing the centre.

2   Players must remember which members of their team are standing next to them.

3   The leader goes into the centre of the square as the spinner. S/he stands still for a minute, facing one of the teams. Players should take note of whether their team is facing the spinner's face, back, right and left side.

4   The spinner spins around. When s/he comes to a stop, s/he yells: 'quick line-up!'

5   The teams must regroup around the spinner in their correct original positions. Every player must be standing in the same relation to the other members of his/her team; every team must be positioned correctly in relation to the spinner.

6   When all the team members are in their correct positions, they yell: 'lined up!'.

7   The first lined-up team is the winner.

Comments

★   All team members should be responsible for helping each other, especially if the game becomes frantic.

Speedy Numbers

Suitability:

Group size: Small / Medium

Procedure

1   The players must sit in a semi-circle and the leader should number them consecutively round the semi-circle from 1 upwards.

2   Number 1 calls another number. Unless that player responds immediately by giving another number, he or she goes to the bottom of the semi-circle and everyone below moves up one place.

3   Players must assume a new number as they move up – for example, if number 6 is sent to the bottom, number 7 becomes number 6, number 8 becomes number 7, and so on.

Comments

★   This game works best if it is played fast.

★   If played with people with walking difficulties, the semi-circle should be kept small. Chairs can also be used. If everyone stands in a strong arc shape walking distances are limited.

★   If you place chairs for people with walking difficulties, remember that wheelchair users cannot play. You could, therefore, split the group into smaller groups accordingly.

What Use is This?

Group size: Small / Medium / Large

Procedure

1   Everyone sits in a circle.

2   An object is placed in the middle (e.g. a shoe) and everyone has to think of as many uses as they can of the ordinary object.

3   Going around the circle, each person gives one use in turn.

4   When someone doesn't give a use, s/he drops out of the game.

5   The game continues until only one player is left.

Comments

★   In order that blind people can take part the object should be verbally introduced at the beginning.

www.ingramcontent.com/pod-product-compliance
Ingram Content Group UK Ltd.
Pitfield, Milton Keynes, MK11 3LW, UK
UKHW050310180625
459797UK00008B/287